Allergy Free

Fast Effective Drug-free Relief for Allergies

Allergy Diet

Allergy Treatments

Allergy Remedies

Natural Allergy Relief

By John McArthur and Cheri Merz

Copyright © 2013 – Natural Health Magazine

Warning

All treatment of any medical condition (without exception) must always be done under supervision of a qualified medical professional. The fact that a substance is "natural" does not necessarily mean that it has no side effects or interaction with other medications.

Medical professionals are qualified and experienced to give advice on side effects and interactions of all types of medication.

Table of Contents

Introduction

Allergies—the runny nose, itchy, red eyes, hacking cough, hives or worse—virtually no individual living in the post-Industrial Age world today is free of sensitivities or allergies and their unfortunate side effects. About 1 in 3 people in the western hemisphere now suffer some form of food intolerance, and as more become aware of the issue, more are coming forward with their own sensitivities. As we will see later, food intolerances have been shown to exacerbate or initiate sensitivity to other allergens as well. Allergies from external sources, i.e., allergens that you take in with every breath you take or with which you come into physical contact, are also widespread. They range in type from natural substances such as grass, flowering plant or tree pollens and animal hair to the more than 3500 food and product additives in use today, to toxins from industrial air and water pollution. The average person is exposed to more than 14kg of toxins each year, through their skin alone.

Allergies develop as a response to constant exposure to foreign substances that your body recognizes as threats, whether they are indeed dangerous or not. It is no wonder that allergies are on the rise - we simply cannot get away from repeated exposure to some of the substances that are most likely to cause them. In a cycle of bad becoming worse, the more your body reacts to allergens, the more stress is put on your system, causing more and more breakdowns to occur. In extremely sensitive individuals, you will find not-so-rare cases of allergy to modern life itself. Fortunately, there are several ways to both avoid developing allergies and to retrain your system to stop recognizing some substances as threats.

Types of Allergies

There are four main sources, or types of allergies. By far the most prevalent are food allergies, followed by environmental factors in the form of inhalants, contactants and injectants. We will discuss each in more detail below. For now, let us define each of them. Food allergies are those reactions to food substances that you ingest or in some rare cases merely brush against or otherwise make contact. Inhalants are substances that enter your system through your nasal passages in particular, although persons who inhale through their mouths are also susceptible in that way. Contactants are substances that you touch, brush against, or that your skin contacts in fabrics or in other ways, usually causing a reaction in the skin. Injectants are substances that are introduced below your skin, such as insect bites or stings and some medications.

Food Allergies

Most people faced with an adverse reaction to a food or other substance will identify it as an allergy. In fact, it could be a sensitivity, an intolerance or a reaction to a toxic or poisonous substance. Although the symptoms might be the same, the causes are somewhat different. An allergy is essentially an immune reaction, an intolerance is rather a sign that you are unable to digest a particular food and of course a toxic reaction is to a substance that is going to make anyone sick or in extreme cases cause death—cyanide gas, for example. As we discuss allergies, we will touch on these other conditions as well.

At the heart of the matter, allergies develop when a substance enters one of your essential bodily function systems that either does not belong there, or is there too often. Thus, there are three main types of allergies, roughly distributed as half food allergies and sensitivities and the rest 'other', or inhalants, injectants and contactants together.

Food allergies and sensitivities also fall into three major groups: those that are common to the very young because of immature digestive systems, those that develop over years of over-exposure, and those that are a result of 'leaky gut syndrome', wherein a compromised digestive tract allows partially digested food particles to enter the blood stream. As we will see, the latter can cause all kinds of havoc; however, let us take the three in order.

Childhood Food Allergy

Probably the most common allergies that appear at a very young age are those to cow's milk and to peanuts. Everyone has heard of a baby whose mother is not nursing for one reason or another becoming very colicky, failing to gain weight or having other problems because its formula is not correct for its young system. In fact, these symptoms can often develop in breast-fed babies too, in response to something the mom is ingesting regularly that does not agree with baby's little tummy. However, it is most common for a baby who is formula-fed to be started on a formula containing cow's milk.

As a whole, western hemisphere countries and particularly the US have traditionally used cow's milk, even long after any other immature animal would have stopped nursing from its mother and begun relying on the food the adults consume. Whether the continuation of that tradition is because 'we have always done it' or because of the dairy lobby in the US, we are raised to believe that milk, specifically cow's milk, is good for us and 'builds strong bones' or 'does a body good'. Children growing up post-Depression were fed formula consisting of sweetened whole cow's milk, and though the industry has come a long way in removing some substances, adding others and making the whole thing more convenient by powdering it to be mixed with water, the fact remains that cow's milk is evolved to nourish baby cattle—not humans. The result is that some baby humans, given repeated exposure to substances within the formula that do not fit baby's needs, quickly develop a life-long sensitivity or allergy to dairy products.

Nor are formulas using some other types of protein exempt from the problem. We have known of babies who are allergic to every type of formula, including soy, rice and milk from other animals. No doubt, the problem is exacerbated because babies take no other nourishment for at least six weeks after birth, resulting in over-exposure. Although goat's or sheep's milk is often touted as the least likely to result in an allergy, the Mayo Clinic advises that this is not the case, because these milks also contain the proteins that cause the problem. Instead, manufacturers are now producing hypoallergenic formulas, some of which use milk that has had the proteins broken down (hydrolyzed) and perhaps further treated using heat or filtering. Depending on the level of processing, these formulas are either classified as partially or extensively hydrolyzed. This is not to be confused with partially-hydrogenated. Other formulas are built, from the ground up so to speak, from individual amino acids, the building blocks of proteins.

There are seven other foods that, along with milk, are responsible for 90% of childhood allergies: eggs, peanuts, wheat, soy, tree nuts (like walnuts, Brazil nuts, and cashews), fish (such as tuna, salmon, and cod), and shellfish (like lobster, shrimp, and crab). The best way to avoid sensitivity, which is often outgrown as the child's digestive system matures, is to avoid giving very young children any food containing these items. Since children often outgrow sensitivity to these foods if they avoid them after an initial reaction, they could actually represent food intolerance rather than allergy.

No matter the cause, if your child exhibits any of the symptoms of food allergy (trouble breathing, swelling of the face or lips, or severe vomiting or diarrhea after eating) you must call 911 right away. A child's airway can close in a matter of minutes, so calling your doctor or driving the child to the emergency room yourself is not an option; you need paramedics on the scene immediately.

Food Allergy in Older Children or Adults

Anyone can develop an allergy to any food at any time, and the reasons for that are more fully explained in the next section, Causes of Allergies. Briefly, though, it is not uncommon for a food that you have enjoyed for years to begin sensitizing you gradually until an immune response develops. As often as not, these gradual onsets of allergies are in response to a food that you eat frequently, causing over-exposure to the allergenic components within it.

Food allergy symptoms range from a tolerable histamine response after ingesting the food to life-threatening anaphylactic shock after merely touching it or raising it to one's lips. If you have a food allergy, you must become proficient at asking questions and reading food labels, although only the most common eight allergens (the same as previously listed for childhood allergies) are required to be listed on warning labels in the US. If your allergy is severe, you may also be well advised to carry an Epi-pen or wear a medical alert bracelet in case of inadvertent exposure to the allergen.

Let us take milk or dairy allergy as an example of why you must ask questions when dining out or as a guest in someone else's home. Without reading the labels of every ingredient, you can never know when milk products are present in other foods.

Hidden sources of milk include whey and casein (milk proteins), any ingredient spelled with the prefix "lact-" — such as lactose and lactate, candies such as chocolate, nougat and caramel, fat-replacement products, such as Simplesse, protein powders, artificial butter flavor, artificial cheese flavor and hydrosolate. Naturally, baked goods may include milk, as may processed breakfast cereals. Even such unlikely foods as canned tuna may contain milk proteins.

Develop the habit of asking when you dine out whether your food contains butter or was dipped in milk before cooking or has cheese as an ingredient of the topping—anything you can think of with regard to the dish you are ordering—and apply these concepts to any other food allergy you have; it could save your life. It is better to endure the momentary embarrassment of closely questioning the wait staff than to suffer a potentially life-threatening reaction to your food.

Be sure also that the server you ask for information actually asks the chef. Research for this book turned up a story about a man who questioned the server about peanut products in the recipe of the dish he was ordering at a Chinese restaurant. Assured that there were none, the man ordered the dish and immediately began experiencing symptoms of anaphylactic shock. As his airway was shutting down, family called 911 and an ambulance was dispatched, but unfortunately, the man died before treatment was able to help him. As it turned out, unbeknownst to the server, peanut butter had been added to the recipe for egg rolls to enhance the flavor. Since no restaurant or individual can possibly be aware of everything that might cause a reaction, it is up to the individual with a severe allergy to protect his own life by asking the right questions of the right people...i.e., the people who are actually preparing the food.

Leaky-Gut Syndrome

Leaky-gut syndrome is not a medical diagnosis at all, but a term that has come to be used by both alternative and traditional medical doctors to describe a set of symptoms for which the cause is not known. As with any illness that involves failure of a body's system, we can describe the failure and how it causes the symptoms, but occasionally we cannot immediately determine why the failure happens. Such is the case with leaky gut syndrome. First described by alternative practitioners and only recently beginning to be recognized by MDs, it is poorly understood. "We don't know a lot but we know that it exists," says Linda A. Lee, MD, a gastroenterologist and director of the Johns Hopkins Integrative Medicine and Digestive Center. "In the absence of evidence, we don't know what it means or what therapies can directly address it."

Evidence is accumulating and even traditional medical practitioners are beginning to recognize that leaky gut syndrome is a real condition that affects the lining of the intestines. The theory is that leaky gut syndrome (also called increased intestinal permeability), is the result of damage to the intestinal lining, although there may be any of several causes for that damage. When damaged, the intestine is less able to protect the internal environment as well as to filter needed nutrients and other biological substances. Some bacteria and their toxins, incompletely digested proteins and fats, and waste not normally absorbed may consequently "leak" out of the intestines into the blood stream. This in turn triggers an autoimmune reaction, leading to gastrointestinal problems such as abdominal bloating, excessive gas and cramps, fatigue, food sensitivities, joint pain, skin rashes, and IBS. All of these conditions, unfortunately, can also be caused by other agents, so that the diagnosis can be quite challenging.

With regard to development of allergies, the theory is that whatever causes the unusual permeability of the intestines allows partially digested food particles to enter the bloodstream, where they are recognized as foreign bodies by the immune system. As a result, the immune response that is the heart of the allergy occurs throughout the body, mimicking or perhaps even being responsible for autoimmune disorders such as Crohn's Disease or fibromyalgia. Treatment is largely experimental at this time, since the causes are not clearly understood. Although doctors do have treatment options, there have been no scientific long-term studies, so results of treatments are anecdotal and not necessarily true for all sufferers.

Inhalants

Sensitivity and allergy to inhalants can be subtle, such as a catch in your throat when you breathe in a certain aroma to life-threatening anaphylaxis and everything in between. While most people experience that catch in the throat after inhaling, say, ammonia, some are sensitive to perfumes, essential oils and scents in everything from air fresheners and candles to dryer sheets and laundry detergent. The key to determining whether you are experiencing an allergic response rather than response to toxic fumes or just a smell you find unpleasant is to classify your symptoms objectively. Does your nose run or do your eyes water? The cause is likely to be either toxic fumes or an allergy—and most people are aware of what fumes in and around households and other public places might be toxic. Ammonia, toluene and chlorine, all toxic in concentration, come to mind as common substances used in cleaning solutions. Breathing these fumes too closely will interfere with your respiration and you are soon driven away from the source. However, if the response is triggered by the scent of a candle or air freshener, you are more likely to be allergic to it. If you do not like the smell but no physical reaction comes from it, then it is merely a personal preference.

Animal dander is also frequently an allergen that enters your body as inhaled particles. Allergy to animals can either be because of inhalants or contactants, and sometimes both. Most people who have animal allergies are sensitive to only one or two types of animals rather than all of them. Animal lovers who find themselves allergic to dogs might consider a cat, or vice versa. Hairless animals also have dander or deposit saliva on their skin when cleaning themselves, or secrete oils to which some people might be allergic. Even fish in an aquarium or bowl may subject the owner to allergens when cleaning the container.

Certain inhalants, such as the ever-present but largely invisible air pollution surrounding large cities, may either be odorless or you may have developed a tolerance for the odor such that you no longer consciously smell it. It is even more frustrating to find yourself with symptoms that indicate allergy but with no perceptible cause.

Injectants

Technically, this class of foreign substance most often has to do with the poisons of insect stings and bites, which you usually receive in such small doses that only a mild itch or reddening occurs. It is when your reaction to the sting or bite is extreme, often causing a serious case of hives or anaphylactic shock, that you would say you are allergic to the toxin. Frequently it is a case of receiving several stings or bites within a few moments, such as when a swarm of bees attacks, that causes an allergy to develop. Unfortunately, this can occur so rapidly that the very first allergic response may result in death. If you have ever developed even a mild case of hives or found yourself gasping for breath after receiving stings or bites, it is imperative to carry emergency epinephrine when you are out-of-doors.

Another source of injected allergens is medication that is hypodermically delivered. In some cases, the medication is toxic and is introduced to combat an even more dangerous illness. It is again when the reaction is extreme, beyond that which most people experience in response to the toxin, that it would be identified as an allergy. An example would be a pain medication that makes most people drowsy and perhaps a little queasy. The person who reacts with violent, projectile vomiting to any amount of the same medication would be said to be allergic to it.

Contactants

This is another class of allergens that consists of both natural substances and those that have been artificially manufactured. Natural allergens include plant fibers such as wool, other animal hair or fur, oils from certain plants (including the toxic oils of poison ivy, oak and sumac) and metals, most frequently nickel or precious metals that have been strengthened with nickel, such as silver and gold jewelry. Other contactants that may cause allergic response include ingredients of soaps, detergents and cosmetics—anything with which your skin comes in frequent contact. Symptoms of this type of allergy are most often rashes, although other symptoms such as hives or infections may occur.

Major Allergy Symptoms and Treatment

Although we have described a few common allergy symptoms and will devote a future section to treatment, we suggest you use this guide arranged by body location to be aware of common symptoms affecting you, the potential severity, and what to do if a symptom is intolerable. This list is not comprehensive, but covers the most common situations.

Eyes

What - Redness, Swelling, Itching, Watering

Allergen - Airborne irritants such as smoke, pollen, industrial pollutants, dust, pet dander

What to Do - Avoid scratching the area, which can lead to infection. A cool compress may provide immediate relief. Your doctor may be able to prescribe topical medication in the form of eye drops or ointment.

Nose

What - Runny nose, Sneezing, Congestion, Sinus headaches, Bloody nose, Infections

Allergen – Airborne irritants such as smoke, pollen, industrial pollutants, dust, pet dander

What to Do - These symptoms can be treated for immediate relief with nasal sprays or over-the-counter antihistamines.*

Severe reactions that lead to bloody nose or infections should be reported to your doctor, to make sure that nothing more serious is at fault.

Mouth

What – Itching in mouth, swelling of tongue and lips

Allergen – Food allergens

What to Do – Avoidance of allergen, emergency epinephrine

Chest/Throat

What – Coughing, Wheezing, Inflammation of bronchial tubes, Tightness of the chest, Mucous buildup, Drop in blood pressure, Anaphylactic shock

Allergen – Airborne irritants, Ingested allergens Food allergens

What to Do – For minor symptoms, drinking a hot beverage such as tea may stop the histamine response. For more severe symptoms, inhalers may be prescribed.* For the most severe symptom, anaphylactic shock, seek emergency treatment.

Stomach/GI Tract

What – Vomiting, diarrhea, abdominal cramps and pain

Allergen – Food allergens

What to Do – Avoidance of allergen

Skin

What – Hives, Rashes, Itchiness, Blisters, Swelling

Allergen – Food allergens, environmental substances such as chemicals, insect bites

What to Do – For mild symptoms or a localized reaction such as to an insect bite, a soothing ointment or gel should be sufficient.

Although several folk remedies purported to draw out the poison or allergen exist, be sure to research their efficacy before using them, as they can be counterproductive.

Food allergies tend to cause systemic skin reactions over a large area. Depending on the severity, medical treatment may be necessary. Some sensitized individuals will react with anaphylactic shock to an insect bite or sting or a severe food allergy; these individuals should have an Epi-pen on hand at all times.

Systemic

What – All of the above

Allergen – Usually caused by toxic overload; see section on Toxic Overload for full discussion

What to Do - Avoidance of all pertinent allergens is the only sure way to gain relief from system-wide allergic response.

*There is some controversy between traditional medicine, which seeks usually to treat symptoms first with medications, and natural medicine, which maintains that the symptoms are serving an essential purpose and should be relieved only through natural methods while the cause is determined and corrected. In the case of allergic rhinitis, overuse of nasal sprays and OTC antihistamines can often lead to a rebound effect, leaving the patient worse off than before. Likewise, patients often misuse inhalers and could be better served by desensitization or other methods of coping with allergy. Avoid long-term use of these medications as described on the usage labels, and seek medical attention if acute symptoms last longer than two weeks. Long-term use of OTC medications should also be under a doctor's supervision.

A word about anaphylactic shock or anaphylaxis: We have mentioned this condition several times, so a definition and more complete explanation are warranted. Anaphylaxis occurs when a person is exposed to an allergen and as a result, the bronchial tubes become inflamed and swollen, constricting the airway. If the reaction is severe enough, the airway can become completely blocked, which results in death if not treated immediately. When signs of anaphylaxis begin, seek emergency medical attention immediately. This severe reaction will not go away on its own.

Causes of Allergies

All allergies are caused by an immune response of the body toward a foreign substance. The mechanism for this response is actually quite fascinating, as it demonstrates how our bodies are self-repairing mechanisms under normal circumstances. An allergen is a protein that the body evaluates and judges to be foreign and therefore dangerous. Upon exposure, the body goes to work to defend against this invader by alerting the immune system that an antigen is present. Thus alerted, the immune system releases specific antibodies to deactivate the antigen, in the form of one or more immunoglobulin proteins designated IgG, IgA, IgM, IgD and IgE. IgE is the immunoglobulin protein most involved in the response to environmental allergens, while IgG is more often involved in the response to food allergies.

Next, mast cells, which produce the allergic response, are activated. The antibody protein signals the mast cells to produce histamine and at least 28 other chemicals that are responsible for the symptoms you experience. As this happens, the antibody proteins attach themselves to the antigens like a peg fitting into the correct hole. There are a number of sizes and shapes of each antibody protein that are specific to each type of allergen. Typically, IgE-mediated allergic response is generally immediate upon exposure to the allergen; at least after sensitization has occurred in the individual, while IgG-mediated response can take up to 72 hours after exposure.

Delayed-response allergies can appear up to 72 hours after exposure to the allergen. These responses are often associated with IgG immunoglobulin antibodies, and might present as other illnesses, leading the sufferer to misdiagnose the symptoms or not believe they are associated with an allergy. Typical symptoms of delayed allergies are lethargy, attention deficit disorder, hyperactivity, itchy skin, mood swings, fatigue, insomnia or inflammation in joints or other tissues. These symptoms are often attributed to one of the mysterious illnesses in the chronic fatigue syndrome/fibromyalgia spectrum or any of several autoimmune disorders. In fact, up to 80 different medical conditions have been associated with IgG immunoglobulin responses to food allergies. If these symptoms sound familiar and you have been diagnosed with arthritis, asthma, insomnia, psoriasis or any other hard-to-manage chronic illness, it might be worth your while to begin keeping a careful food diary and noting when flare-ups of your condition occur within 72 hours of ingesting a food that commonly causes allergic response.

The most common cause of environmental allergies are the pollens of trees, weeds, flowers and grasses, as well as dust mites, molds, tobacco smoke and pet dander. Playing an increasingly important role, however, are the thousands of chemicals that surround modern man. We now spend up to 90% of our time indoors, with many artificial substances from carpet fibers to paint exuding VOCs (volatile organic compounds) constantly. Despite efforts to reduce the chemical gasses to which we are exposed, the fact is that they are many times higher now than at any other time in the history of humankind. Chemical sensitivities are a relatively new phenomenon simply because people were not exposed to so many chemicals in past times. Nowadays, evidence is accumulating that as many as 1000 new chemicals are introduced to our environment each year.

As early as the 1980s, scientists began using the acronym SBS (for sick building syndrome) to describe a cluster of symptoms experienced by office workers when high-efficiency buildings that re-circulated the same stale air, pathogens and chemical fumes, began making dozens ill at a time. With perfect irony, the phenomenon was brought to the attention of the general public when the offices of the Environmental Protection Agency were reported by CBS to be environmentally unsafe for workers. As high profile and indignation rousing as these facts are, however, food allergies are by far the more prevalent cause of illness and in fact have been shown to exacerbate the development of environmental allergies.

Food allergies are defined as abnormal or adverse immunological responses to foods that others can eat with no reaction. The operative phrase however is 'immunological responses'. Food allergies must be distinguished from non-allergic reactions to foods caused by enzyme deficiency, poor digestion or food poisoning as well as toxic reactions that anyone would experience if they ingested a toxic substance. According to Alternative Medicine, The Definitive Guide (second edition) the USDA estimates that only about 15% of the population reacts to foods, but that of those only 1.5% experience true, immunologically-mediated reactions. The rest are a result of food intolerance, a broad category that includes food poisoning and toxicity, anaphylactoid reactions and other mediator-release reactions, pharmacologic reactions (reactions to drugs), metabolic food reactions and food idiosyncratic reactions. The latter refers to food sensitivities for which the biological mechanism is not well understood, and includes such reactions as hyperactivity in children as a response to certain food additives or sugar, headaches in response to the food additive MSG and even celiac disease, a reaction to gluten-containing foods. Metabolic food reactions include adverse reactions to foods that contain certain substances for which the individual's body lacks the enzyme to break it down, like lactose intolerance or phenylketonuria.

This is not to say that these disorders are less important than food allergies, as they can have serious consequences ranging from failure to thrive to mental retardation to death. It is very important to distinguish between food allergies and food intolerances simply because the methods we will discuss in later sections to alleviate certain allergies will not help food intolerances based in genetic defect. It is also important to realize that traditional allergy testing may not reveal food sensitivities or intolerances that are not immunologically mediated.

Finally, you should be aware of cross-reactivity. If you determine, for example, that you are allergic to shrimp, chances are that you are also allergic to other types of shellfish, such as crabs, lobster and crayfish.

The foregoing information is widely recognized by both traditional and alternative practitioners. There are a number of additional theories that alternative practitioners have espoused, and some of them are beginning to be studied or recognized by researchers and MDs. The following sections explore these theories.

Imbalanced Immune System

Dr. Leon Chaitow, a highly respected naturopathic and osteopath from London, England is quoted in Alternative Medicine (ibid) as having found that a number of factors negatively impact the immune function. Included are increased toxic burden due to pollution in all its forms, disturbance of immune systems through repeated childhood and adult vaccinations and immunizations, and damage to healthy intestinal flora due to overreliance on antibiotics and steroids, particularly birth control pills. Because allergies by definition are immunologically mediated, it stands to reason that any factor that impairs immune function can set you up for the development of allergies. In particular, the over-use of antibiotics and resultant elimination of beneficial intestinal flora so confuses your immune system that the rebound effect can be worse than the original illness. System-wide candidiasis, for example, has been identified as the culprit in any number of chronic illnesses, and is given free reign when beneficial flora are not present.

Repetitive Diet/Food Addictions

Surveys show that the diets of allergy patients typically consist of 30 or fewer foods, leading to the conclusion that a monotonous diet leads to over-exposure of the immune system to these foods, and in turn to development of an allergy. Whether this is the case or whether the foods involved are typically those that are most allergenic, it again makes sense that a variety of foods will allow the individual less exposure to those that might cause allergies. Charles Gableman, M.D., a former practitioner of environmental medicine in California, goes so far as to say that, "The likelihood of having an allergic reaction to any food is directly proportionate to how often a person eats it." This theory also ties into the theory that some foods are addictive and that we are likely to be allergic to the very foods to which we are addicted. The fact that we may not experience adverse reactions to the food until it is withdrawn is attributed to a phenomenon called 'masking', which means that consuming the food hides the allergic response. Based on the definitions of allergy vs. food intolerance, it seems more likely that at least the latter or possibly both the theories under discussion here are actually describing food intolerances rather than true, immunologically mediated allergies.

Barrier Function Default

This theory espouses the fact that certain of our bodily systems are designed as barriers to keep the outside out. For example, digestion is designed to break down complex food molecules into their component nutrients that the body can put to use. Any malfunction of digestion, whether caused by illness, medication, genetic deficiency or other agency, can lead to improper digestion and the potential of leaky gut syndrome. Although, as we have previously mentioned, this is not a medical diagnosis, the mechanism for the condition causing allergies is easily described and understood. Through a breakdown of the digestive process, partially digested food particles enter the bloodstream and are treated as antigens as in the above description of the process. Causes for digestive malfunction can include excessive alcohol consumption, viral, fungal or bacterial infections, parasites, use of non-steroidal anti-inflammatory drugs (NSAIDS), antibiotics, excessive stress and radiation.

Likewise, the mucous coating the lining of nasal passages and lungs is designed to trap and keep out large particles that would be foreign to respiratory function. Cilia, small hair-like organs, move the particles mixed with mucous to the upper throat (pharynx) where they are expelled by coughing or swallowed and destroyed by stomach acid and digestive enzymes. Environmental irritants, dry air and some medications can damage the mucous membranes and allow the particles instead to enter the bloodstream where once again they are recognized as antigens.

Finally, the skin is the third barrier, and compromising it can also allow the introduction of allergens. Dry or damaged skin that comes into frequent contact with fabrics, dyes, chemicals in laundry detergent and other household chemicals, cosmetics, perfume and aftershave products allows sensitization most frequently. Even lotions or topical medications can be a factor, and perspiration or heat that causes the blood vessels near the skin to dilate and increase absorption can exacerbate the problem. Other factors affecting absorption through the skin include those that impair the skin's repair functions, such as deficiency of water or essential fatty acids, hormonal irregularities, ultraviolet radiation and stress.

In considering this theory, we must wonder which comes first, the malfunction of the barrier, or the introduction of the attacker, which could cause the breach from within. Nevertheless, particularly with regard to the digestion, it is certainly a good idea to do everything in our power to maintain the barriers that Nature has given us for our internal defenses.

Toxic Overload

We bear an enormous toxic burden as a result of living in airtight houses, in cities where the air is polluted with auto exhaust and industrial emissions, eating foods that have been doused with fertilizer or insecticide and possibly genetically engineered, and all the other perils of modern life. Our immune systems were not designed to have to keep up with the overwhelming onslaught of these toxins, and are therefore weakened by doing so. By the very nature of how allergies develop, a weakened immune system means more allergies. In fact, this cause may not even belong in the 'alternative theory' category, as more and more environmental physicians with 'M.D.' behind their names get on the bandwagon to warn of the dangers we face. Ultimately, an overburdened immune system allows all types of allergies to develop, and in extreme cases, the result is described as allergy to modern life. While many of the allergy treatments we will discuss in the appropriate section may relieve individual allergies, a syndrome of allergy to modern life can only be treated by removing all synthetic substances, allergenic foods and airborne allergens from the individual's environment.

Diagnosis/Testing for Allergies

The first order of business when you suspect you are sensitive to, allergic to or intolerant of a substance is to begin keeping a diary of your reactions and what you have been doing, eating and drinking for the 72 hours prior to the response. Of course, if the response is severe you will probably be experiencing an immediate reaction and should seek immediate medical attention. On the other hand, if your suspected sensitivity or allergy is to a substance you can easily avoid and your symptoms are minor, it may not be necessary to formally test and diagnose the allergy at all. The degree to which you are inconvenienced or made ill by the allergy will probably be your best guide as to whether you will seek a diagnosis or merely employ some of the desensitization and avoidance techniques we will discuss in later sections.

There are surprisingly few methods of testing for allergies, and some are more effective for diagnosing certain types of allergens than others. We will explore each in detail.

Skin Tests

There are three main types of skin testing, all of which primarily identify IgE-medicated allergic responses. They are the skin prick or scratch test, the intradermal test, and the skin patch test.

Skin Prick/Scratch Test

This is the conventional method for identifying allergens responsible for IgE-mediated allergic responses such as allergic rhinitis, eczema, hives and asthma. Typically, responses such as these are triggered by inhaled allergens such as pollen, mold, dust mites or animal dander. Unfortunately, this type of test is only about 15% effective in detecting food allergies according to one researcher.

The skin test procedure is very simple: the doctor lightly scratches or uses a fine needle to lightly prick the skin in a pre-determined pattern. Small dilutions of the suspected allergens are then introduced carefully to each damaged skin area so that the allergen can enter the body. If a wheal (a reddish inflammation similar to a mosquito bite) develops within 20 minutes, an allergy to the substance is confirmed. It may require several sessions to test for every allergen, with the most common ones being tested first. Here is where your diary may come in handy, to suggest a more efficient order of testing than if you were to simply go to your allergist and ask to be tested for all known allergens.

Intradermal Test

This test is performed when the skin prick test does not show a reaction to the allergen, but it is still suspected as the cause of an individual's reaction. The intradermal test is more sensitive than the skin prick test, but is also responsible for more false positive results. In this test, the allergen solution is injected into the skin.

Skin Patch Test

This test is used to detect contact dermatitis, a type of allergy or sensitivity that causes a rash upon contact. To perform it, the suspected allergen is placed on a pad that is then taped to the person's skin for 24 to 72 hours.

Laboratory Blood Testing

Blood tests may not be as sensitive as skin tests, but for allergies that are not easily determined by skin testing, or for individuals that for some reason cannot have a skin test, several blood tests are available.

IgG ELISA Test

Testing for food allergies can be more challenging than determining environmental allergy responses. Most food allergies are dealt with by IgG antibodies, whereas the traditional skin prick test measures only the IgE-mediated responses. For this reason, many practitioners, particularly those well versed in alternative medicine; consider the ELISA test to be one of the most sensitive and therefore most useful blood tests to detect delayed food allergies. ELISA stands for enzyme-linked immunoserological assay.

To perform this test, a small blood sample is taken from the patient and then delivered within 72 hours to a specialized laboratory that is equipped to process the assay. Here, technicians collect the IgG antibodies within the sample, and place a drop of the serum containing the antibodies into a laboratory testing plate consisting of many tiny depressions or 'wells'. Each of these wells contains a single food or component of food, such as gluten, that are known to be potentially allergenic. A computer then analyzes the samples for reaction to the food. A positive reaction indicates that the specific IgG antibody to that food exists within the sample, and means that an allergic response will occur within the individual's body when that food is ingested, particularly in the presence of leaky gut syndrome.

EIA Test

This test, similar to ELISA, measures IgE antibodies that mediate most environmental allergies.

Other Blood Tests

Other lab testing methods, such as radioallergosorbent testing (RAST) or an immunoassay capture test (ImmunoCAP, UniCAP, or Pharmacia CAP), may be used to provide more information. Similar to the ELISA and EIA tests, these tests use laboratory methods to isolate antibodies and test them against known allergens for reaction.

Challenge Testing

Because skin testing is not particularly useful for food allergies and certain medications, an allergist might recommend a challenge test for these substances. To perform the test, a very small amount of a potential allergen is inhaled or ingested by the patient. It is critical that this type of test be supervised by a doctor in a medical setting where emergency procedures are in place, as even a small amount of a substance that is ingested or inhaled can cause anaphylactic shock and death in a highly susceptible patient.

Electrodermal Screening (EDS)

Although few clinical studies have been done to test the effectiveness of this method, it is widely used in Europe to screen for both food and environmental allergies, and to determine the proper remedy. In a couple of very small clinical trials done in the late 1990s, the test was 82% and 96% accurate, respectively, in differentiating between specific allergens and in discriminating between allergenic and non-allergenic substances, leading researchers to state that it is a reliable method for detecting allergy triggers. At this time, the FDA has not approved any device of this nature for marketing in the US, has warned several manufacturers to stop making false claims, and has disciplined some practitioners for their use and claims for this type of testing due to lack of clinical trials supporting the claims.

To perform this test, the doctor introduces a small current of electricity at specific acupuncture points on the patient. The doctor then introduces various allergens into the circuitry, enabling the physician to determine any change in the patient's reaction to the current. In this type of testing, the circuitry is also used to deliver treatment doses when an allergy reaction is determined. The full battery of tests can be completed in one hour.

Applied Kinesiology

George Goodheart, D.C., of Detroit, MI, first developed the theory and study of the relationship between muscle dysfunction or weakness and related organ or gland dysfunction. Research for this book has turned up no clinical studies of the practice of applied kinesiology, not to be confused with kinesiology (the scientific study of the movement of the human body). Nevertheless, alternative medical practitioners, particularly chiropractors in this case, believe that with regard to allergies, when an allergen contacts an allergic person, its energetic properties will block the flow of energy within the body, resulting in weakened muscles. To perform the test, the patient holds a glass vial containing the allergen in the less-dominant hand while raising the opposing arm to a 90° angle at the shoulder with the elbow straight. While the patient resists, the practitioner then pushes lightly on the raised arm, down toward the patient's side. If the patient has little resistance to the pressure, the weak muscle response indicates an allergy or sensitivity to the substance in the vial.

Diagnosis and Testing Controversy

As you might imagine after reading the foregoing descriptions, there is a great deal of controversy between conventional and alternative practitioners regarding the efficacy of each other's methods. In fact, there is also some controversy among members of each community. For example, the American Academy of Allergy, Asthma & Immunology (AAAAI) believes that IgG testing is not useful or effective despite other M.D.s recommending it. Nor does AAAAI approve of applied kinesiology, electro dermal screening and several other frankly alternative and mysterious methods that we have not covered. It is up to you as a well-informed individual to determine the best course of action when you are seeking the cause of a reaction that is not easily understood. Despite the Western bias toward what we call conventional medicine, plenty of anecdotal evidence exists that alternative methods can be effective, even when we do not understand the scientific basis that would explain why they are effective. We would not necessarily recommend that someone with a severe or life-threatening reaction start with methods that have not been scientifically proven; nevertheless, we could cite many cases where individuals have had to become their own diagnosticians, demand certain tests or take charge of their own treatment because science does not have all the answers.

Allergy Prevention

As well understood as the mechanisms of allergy response and other sensitivities are, medical science is still in the discovery phase as to why in some cases our immune systems become over-sensitive and decide to attack what would otherwise be innocuous proteins. Why, for example, are there more allergy sufferers in the US than in Europe, where the cities are as heavily air-polluted or more so than comparable US cities? Could it really be, as some alternative practitioners have suggested, that our reliance on antibiotics and early-childhood vaccinations are actually counterproductive with regard to allergies? How are we to resolve the fact that without vaccinations, children are left open to serious illness, but with them may be left open to life-threatening asthma attacks? For that matter, what is the right thing to do when we know that mothers who have serious allergies can pass on the antigens and antibodies to their newborns through breast milk, when we know that otherwise breast milk is the most beneficial for baby's nutrition and immune function?

Aside from these difficult decisions, the old adage 'an ounce of prevention is worth a pound of cure' is particularly apt with regard to allergies. The best practices for allergy prevention will be presented in this section, along with cautions and other considerations.

Allergy Prevention for Children

Breast Feed Your Infant

Long-term research has proven that the best way to equip your newborn to cope with assaults from illness and allergy is to feed him with mother's breast milk exclusively for the first few months of life. It is the only substance that was designed by evolution to be the perfect food for immature human digestive systems. That said, what of the evidence that even newborns fed exclusively on breast milk can exhibit signs of food allergy? Anecdotal evidence would suggest that if the mother removes foods from her diet to which she and baby both react, baby's sensitivities would clear up relatively quickly. Once again, the best way to determine to what the baby might be reacting is to keep a food diary along with a diary of baby's reactions. There is no scientific evidence that allergies are inherited, while there is plenty of such evidence that mom's immunities are passed through her milk. Significantly, IgG antibodies are passed through the placenta to the developing fetus' blood supply. The best way to avoid these unintended consequences is for mom to address her allergies and sensitivities before becoming pregnant, and to avoid allergens while pregnant and nursing.

Some mothers find themselves unable or, more rarely unwilling, to breast-feed for one reason or another. If you find yourself in this situation, certainly there are nutritionally adequate formulas on the market. We would suggest you start with a hypoallergenic formula to avoid development of allergies to the ingredients of other formulas.

Introduce Solid Foods Later

The longer you can delay introducing solid foods to your infant, the more mature her digestive system will be and the less likely to develop food allergies or sensitivities. Several decades ago, it was common to breastfeed exclusively until the infant was six months old, up to one year. However, with more and more moms attempting to work full- or part-time while pumping breast milk, it seems that it is less practical, and that baby is demanding something more filling at an earlier and earlier age. Some mothers introduce baby cereals as young as six weeks, either because baby does not seem to be satisfied with just breast milk, or in an attempt to induce sleeping through the night. Given the fact that some cereals (wheat, in particular) are among the most allergenic eight foods for children, introducing these foods early is tailor-made for allergy disaster.

If you must introduce solid foods at an early age, avoid at all cost the eight most common allergenic foods, listed in the Types of Allergies: Food Allergies section. Instead, opt for fresh fruits and vegetables, legumes and low-fat proteins such as fish (not shellfish) or chicken. It is best to avoid highly processed foods and prepare your own using a blender designed for the purpose. This will allow you also to limit the sugars, sodium and preservatives that are not particularly healthful for your child and have their own risks for allergies.

Avoid Early Immunization

One of the more controversial recommendations alternative medicine practitioners often make is to avoid vaccinations. Controversial because deaths from the childhood diseases that we typically immunize for in the US have been radically lowered by vaccination, the fact remains that a small but statistically important number of children experience death or irreparable damage from vaccines yearly. If your child is cared for by a conventional medical practitioner, she will likely require you to allow a series of immunization shots starting when your baby is only two months old. Beginning with hepatitis B, a combination diphtheria/tetanus/pertussis, influenza type B and polio, your child may be subjected to an average of up to 21 shots over the first 15 months of her life. Any one of them could trigger an allergic reaction that might range from temporary discomfort and fever to death.

Before you decide that your own child will by no means be subjected to this regimen, consider the fact that 90% of infants infected with hepatitis B will become chronically infected, with higher lifetime risk of cirrhosis and hepatocellular carcinoma, as well as being the largest source of new infections among the general public. Diphtheria, a bacterial disease, causes a thick coating in the back of the throat that can lead to breathing problems, paralysis, heart problems and even death. In the 1920s, prior to the vaccine being developed, it led to 150,000 deaths per year. Although the current risk of diphtheria in the US is very low, approximately 25 cases over the last 20 years, resulting in five deaths, outbreaks in Eastern Europe in the 1990s followed a drop in immunization rates. Nor are we isolated here in the US, as modern travel increasingly makes local outbreaks of any disease a global crisis if the disease is life threatening. Similarly, pertussis, another bacterial disease causes whooping cough so severe that it is hard for an infant to eat, drink or breathe. It can lead to pneumonia, seizures, brain damage and death.

We could go on, but the impact is clear: complete avoidance of immunizations could be just as dangerous as allowing immunizations. The answer may lie in consulting with your child's doctor to delay the immunizations if the risk of infection is small, a compromise that could lower the risk of allergic reaction to the vaccine. If you choose not to have your child vaccinated, understand that the consequences could be not only risk of the illness, but also risk of falling afoul of state and local law or later school requirements. In the case that you feel strongly enough to withstand the social pressure to have your child vaccinated, you might explore obtaining an exemption from local authorities, based on religious, medical or philosophical beliefs.

Remove Allergens from Your Home

To the extent possible, make sure your home is free of air-borne and other environmental allergens. Addressing dust mites, pet dander, molds, smoke, formaldehyde from housing components, paint fumes, etc. before bringing your infant home can protect him from early sensitization to these allergens and can be especially helpful in preventing the development of asthma. Be sure you also test for radon gas, a carcinogenic substance emitted from the earth itself that collects in enclosed areas.

You can reduce exposure to common allergens in your home up to 95% by taking the following precautions:

Whole House

- Do not smoke indoors
- Keep windows closed, especially during 'allergy season' or periods of high wind
- Humidify or de-humidify to achieve optimal relative humidity
- Remove longstanding odors and particulates with an ozone air purifier with no people, animals or plants in the area while the purifier is running
- Maintain clean air with air filters and HEPA vacuum cleaner bags

Bedroom and Nursery

- Eliminate or limit exposure of pets to the bedroom or nursery

- Remove bedroom carpeting or treat with tannic acid to denature allergens

- Remove stuffed animals from the bed or crib

- Wash pillows, blankets and crib bumpers monthly in the hottest water possible

- Use washable organic cotton pillows

- Enclose mattresses in plastic mite-proof covers

Additional Allergy Prevention for Everyone

Many cosmetics and personal care items contain numerous chemicals, perfumes and preservative additives that can trigger allergies. To avoid these, buy the most natural products you can find, or use time-honored substitutes. For example, baking soda was the tooth cleaner of choice before commercial toothpastes became common. For other personal care items, explore the growing number of companies that practice organic and green technologies to produce skin, hair and body care products.

Mold allergies can be prevented by the simple expedient of preventing or remediating the source. Along with maintaining the proper relative humidity in your home, be sure to clean often and regularly all bathrooms, laundry rooms, refrigerators, humidifiers and other appliances that use water. Change furnace and air conditioner filters, particularly evaporative coolers, at appropriate intervals. Make sure your basement is not damp, or take corrective action. In addition, in severe cases, consider avoiding food that might contain mold spores, such as mushrooms, aged cheeses and any leftover food.

Avoid unnecessary damage to your skin by using sunscreen or limiting your exposure to early morning and late afternoon. If you already have allergies that manifest in skin rashes, do not use hair dyes or have tattoos, as these are common triggers.

Opt for substances that are more natural and fewer chemicals in your water, clothing, household furnishings and any other major contributor to your environment. Be aware of local issues in particular, but also of all common coatings, additives and emissions in your surroundings. An example would be when you purchase new clothing. Perhaps the label claims that the item is made from 100% pure cotton, but did you know that there is a substance on most new fabrics called sizing? Cotton rarely causes an allergic reaction itself, but azo dyes, disperse dyes and formaldehyde resins used to give a non-wrinkle finish may cause sensitization. Other natural fibers may be allergenic in and of themselves, wool being a prime example. When you paint or re-carpet your home, choose low-VOC products.

Preventing Allergic Response to Known Allergies

Once you have become sensitized, the question becomes whether you can somehow prevent or avoid the allergic response, especially to environmental factors over which you have no control, such as pollen count. The following tips will help you minimize your exposure to the environmental allergens that make you miserable.

Be Forewarned About High Pollen Counts

Check daily pollen counts on AAAAI's website. Stay indoors or take other appropriate precautions when pollens you are allergic to are present.

Wear a Mask

If you must be exposed to high pollens, for example while gardening or lawn mowing, wear an N25 filter mask (available for about $25 for 20), which will keep pollen out of your nose and mouth.

Wash Your Hair in the Evening

Hair care products can trap pollen, which is then deposited on your pillow where you can inhale it as you sleep. Wash your hair before bed to remove the day's pollen and get a good night's sleep.

Let Go of Stress

A stressful day can increase levels of the stress hormone cortisol, which in turn can exacerbate allergic reactions. Meditate, relax in a warm tub or do any of a myriad of stress-releasing exercises to turn down the cortisol effect.

Keep Your Nose Clean

Pollen sticks to the lining of your nasal passages, according to allergists. You can try a saline sinus rinse, found at any drugstore, to rinse harmful pollen away. If that does not work for you, you can buy a nonprescription herbal nasal spray called NasalCrom (cromolyn sodium) to help prevent allergic reactions in your sinuses.

Banish Dust Mites

Dust mites thrive in environments that are above 70 degrees Fahrenheit and above 50% humidity. Keep your home temperatures in the mid-60's and humidity at the 40-45% level to rid your home of these pests.

Barriers and Boiling

Thwart dust mites also with mattress covers and pillow encasements that are impervious to the miniscule creatures. You do not literally have to boil your bedding, but washing it frequently in the hottest water the fabric can tolerate will also ban the critters.

Outsource Housekeeping

Dusting and vacuuming stir up dust mites and their droppings, both of which are highly allergenic. In addition to using HEPA filters in your vacuum cleaner, hire someone else to do the dusting and vacuuming and stay out of your house for the two hours it takes the particulates to settle.

Try Acupuncture

One theory is that acupuncture reduces levels of stress and stress hormones. In any case, plenty of anecdotal evidence exists that indicates acupuncture can help with allergies.

Pet Grooming

In addition to banning Fido and Missy from the bedroom, have someone take your pets outside for a good brushing every day. Using a comb dipped in distilled water will trap dander. A once-a-month bath for Fido is also necessary, but more often will dry his skin, making the dander problem worse.

Environmental allergens may be ubiquitous, but with a little effort, you can arrange your life to avoid them as much as possible to prevent the allergic reactions. When all else fails, therapies ranging from supplements to steroids are available. We will discuss treatment in a later section.

Foods to Avoid

Along with avoiding the eight most common food allergens, be aware of the cross-reactions that can be triggered by foods that are of similar origins. For example, if you develop an allergy to latex, you could also be sensitive to fruits of similar types of trees, which might include bananas, nectarines, avocados and other trees with sap that has rubber-like properties. The type of allergy at work here is called Oral Allergy Syndrome, and occurs when pollen of one allergen sensitizes you to fruits, vegetables and occasionally nuts from the same family of plant. If you have pollen allergies, you will want to watch for these cross-reactions:

- Ragweed allergy theoretically cross-reacts with bananas and melons, so people with a ragweed allergy might also react to cantaloupe, honeydew or watermelon. Also suspect are tomatoes, Echinacea, zucchini, sunflower seeds, dandelions and chamomile tea.

- Birch pollen allergy sufferers may react to apples, pears, peaches, kiwi, plums, coriander, fennel, parsley, celery, cherries, carrots, hazelnuts, and almonds.

- According to the AAAAI, people with grass allergy may react to peaches, celery, tomatoes, melons, and oranges, according to the AAAAI.

- Mugwort allergies are associated with sensitivity to celery, carrot, spices, melon, apple, hazelnut and chestnut

OAS tends to develop over time with repeated exposure to the primary allergen as well as to the trigger food. Because the reaction can be rapid, coming within half an hour of eating the offending food, and severe (including facial numbness, swelling of the throat and nasal passages leading to airway obstruction and anaphylactic shock), do not eat a food if it has previously given you even minor reactions such as tingling of the tongue, itching or numbness of the lips, tongue or face or swelling of nasal passages or glands in the throat. If it is a favorite food, under close supervision try it cooked, peeled or canned. The proteins that are most reactive are found in the skins of fruits and vegetables, so peeling may eliminate enough of them to allow you to tolerate the food. Cooking, including the heating process used in canning, breaks down those proteins and potentially renders them harmless.

Other types of food allergy or intolerance require you to avoid different foods. If you are allergic to wheat, it is instructive to determine whether it is actually the gluten to which you are sensitive. True celiac disease, in which the patient lacks the enzyme to break down the gluten, is relatively rare. However, immunoglobulin-mediated responses to wheat do occur, and there is growing evidence that some people just feel better if they avoid it. If you suspect you are sensitive to wheat gluten, you will probably want to avoid any gluten-containing grain, including barley and rye in addition to all forms of wheat. Buckwheat is among the gluten-free grains and despite its name is not really wheat.

If you are allergic to any one type of shellfish, you have a 75% chance of being allergic to another or all of them, but there is usually little cross-reactivity to other fish. Avoidance of all types of shellfish is necessary if allergy is a concern, because shellfish allergy accounts for up to 1/3 of all serious allergic reactions. It is a common misconception stemming from the 1970s that shellfish allergy is actually allergy to iodine. There is no evidence that this is the case, nor is there any correlation between shellfish, iodine and radio contrast dyes (used for CT scans and other medical imaging), another common allergy.

Tree nuts (as opposed to peanuts, a legume) are a common allergen, and once again you would want to avoid all tree nuts after developing an allergy to one variety, at least until the extent of the allergic response has been determined. Peanuts are among the most common allergies of all, and despite advice found in research for the section above on childhood allergy, there is some evidence that delaying introduction of peanuts and peanut products to a child's diet has little effect or even contributes to later development of the allergy. It is this type of confusing evidence that makes diagnosing allergies and determining what allergens are at work so difficult.

Most alternative practitioners will also tell you to avoid sugar, mucous-forming foods such as cow's milk and other dairy, refined grains and other highly processed foods. Some will also warn against alcohol, chocolate, tea, coffee, meats and other animal protein, smoked, salted or pickled foods and any foods containing artificial flavorings or coloring. We agree that many of these foods are nutritionally void and some have been shown to be carcinogenic. However, we take exception to eliminating chocolate; one of the great pleasures in life that also has antioxidant properties...unless you are sensitive to it, of course.

Treatment of Allergies

Conventional treatment of allergies begins with conventional testing to determine the type of allergen to which the patient reacts, followed by avoidance of the allergen and symptom relief medications if warranted. Finally, some allergies respond to immunotherapy with desensitization. While the allergy sufferer may be thankful for the relief provided by antihistamines, inhalers and topical creams for rash, none of these treatments provides a cure for the allergy or an expectation of future amelioration of the symptoms. Alternative medicine practitioners believe that the preferred treatment is to attack the problem at the source, by employing various methods that they claim not only will alleviate symptoms, but also eliminate the allergy response in the future. This section discusses each type of medication or method and identifies it as either conventional or alternative.

Epinephrine

Epinephrine is the treatment of choice in an emergency situation involving anaphylactic shock or other severe allergic reaction. Otherwise known as adrenaline, epinephrine is a hormone whose function in the body is as a neurotransmitter. It regulates heart rate, blood vessel and air passage diameter and metabolic shifts, and is a crucial component in the 'fight-or-flight' survival response. Because of its action in dilating air passages and bronchial tissue, patients at risk for anaphylaxis from commonly encountered allergens may be prescribed an auto-injector, sometimes known by one of its trade names, Epi-pen, for emergency use. Adverse reactions to epinephrine are heart palpitations, tachycardia, arrhythmia, anxiety, panic attack, headache, tremor, hypertension, and acute pulmonary edema. The more minor or harmless though uncomfortable reactions are certainly preferable to loss of airway, however, and dissipate rapidly as the immediate effect of the epinephrine wears off.

Antihistamines and Decongestants

Since the origin of uncomfortable allergy symptoms are chemicals called histamines that are produced within the body as an immunological response, medicines that counteract these chemicals are called antihistamines. The numerous varieties are available in tablet, capsule, inhalant, liquid, nasal spray and eye drop form, some by prescription and some over the counter (OTC). All of them work by binding to the same receptors that histamine would bind to, blocking the effect of the histamine, and therefore are more effective when taken before exposure to the allergen. Therefore, some doctors recommend combining the antihistamine with a decongestant, which shrinks swollen tissues and acts on some symptoms for which antihistamines are ineffective. Combination formulas may also prevent mast cells from releasing other chemicals associated with allergy.

Antihistamines can cause many side effects, such as dry mouth, drowsiness, dizziness, nausea and vomiting, restlessness or moodiness (in some children), trouble urinating or not being able to urinate, blurred vision or confusion. Older first-generation antihistamines such as those that go by the brand names Benadryl, Chlor-Trimetron and Tavist tend to cause more side effects than the newer medications. You should always read labels on medications if you are taking other medications, whether OTC or prescribed, as some medicines can interact and either cause a reaction in combination or render one another ineffective. Similarly, decongestants can also cause many of the same side effects and can worsen heart problems.

Steroids

Steroids, also known as corticosteroids, can prevent and treat nasal stuffiness, itchy, runny nose or sneezing due to pollen and other environmental allergies. They can also decrease inflammation and swelling from other types of allergic reactions. Systemic steroids are available in several modes of delivery, but the main issue is that they must be taken regularly, even daily, even when you are not exhibiting any allergy symptoms. In addition, it can take up to two weeks before the full effect of the medication develops.

Steroids can be given in a short course of treatment for some problems with little ill effect, chiefly temporary weight gain, fluid retention and elevated blood pressure. When given orally, systemically and/or for long periods, steroids can produce a number of more serious side effects such as growth suppression, diabetes, and cataracts of the eyes, bone-thinning (osteoporosis) or muscle weakness. Long-term inhalation of steroids for bronchial asthma symptoms can include cough, hoarseness or fungal infection of the mouth

Mast Cell Stabilizers

Since allergy symptoms are a direct result of chemicals released by mast cells, it stands to reason that medications designed to prevent those chemical releases can be used to prevent allergic reactions, especially asthma. These medications also have some anti-inflammatory effect, but typically are not as effective for that purpose as are steroids. An advantage is that the side effects associated with mast cell stabilizers are milder than those of steroids are. They include throat irritation, coughing or skin rashes as well as minor stinging or blurred vision when applied as eye drops. Some specific brands also induce a bad taste, which can be reduced by drinking juice after taking the medicine.

Leukotriene Modifiers

Leukotrienes, like histamines, are chemicals released by mast cells in response to allergens. Leukotriene modifiers block the effects of the substance. Side effects are rare, but may include stomach pain or stomach upset, heartburn, fever, stuffy nose, cough, rash, headache, irritability or behavioral issues.

All of the above medications are available with prescriptions, although some are also available in OTC formulations. We find it ironic that many of the side effects exhibit the same symptoms that the sufferer of allergies is trying to alleviate in the first place. Therefore, the following are non-medical symptom relief suggestions.

OTC saline solutions available as nasal sprays or delivered by nasal rinse devices can relieve mild congestion, loosen mucous and prevent crusting. If you opt for the use of a nasal rinse device (neti-pot), be sure to observe strict sterilization procedures to avoid infection.

Artificial tears, a special formula of saline solution, can relieve red, itchy, watery eyes. Neither this nor the previous product contains any medicine.

Immunotherapy

Immunotherapy, or allergy shots, works by gradually building tolerance to the allergen through introduction of increasing amounts by injection. If you suffer from allergies more than three months of the year, this may be the most effective traditional treatment. Speak to your allergist to learn the potential benefits and cautions for your particular form of allergy.

Alternative and Natural Therapies

Most alternative therapies depend upon avoidance of the allergen and any cross-reactive substances, but also include dietary and supplementation suggestions to strengthen the immune system. It certainly cannot hurt to follow a nutritional plan that includes plenty of fresh, organic nutrient-dense foods. Typically, these include fresh fruits and vegetables, legumes and grains (with the exception of gluten-containing grains for sensitive people) that are not highly processed. Be mindful that if allergens that cause your reactions include those listed as cross-reactive with fruits and vegetables in the Foods to Avoid section, above, you should limit your choices of those items to fruits and vegetables not included in the lists. The next section will list some allergy-friendly foods; i.e., those that either are not highly allergenic or that will provide nutrients that strengthen the immune system in specific ways to avoid allergic reactions.

In addition to proper choices in your diet, some practitioners suggest that a rotation diet can help avoid developing allergies in the first place. The theory is that you not only get a wider variety of nutrients, but also avoid eating any one food too often, thus preventing sensitization. One practitioner advises not eating any one food more often than once every four days, although you might have several servings of it on the day that you do eat it. Eating a wider variety of foods has many other benefits, as well, such as avoiding becoming bored with your food.

While you are choosing these foods, maintaining awareness of the so-called Stone Age diet can also be useful. This diet depends on the theory that our digestive system has developed very slowly, and at this point in evolution has not progressed past the Paleolithic era, when people ate fish, vegetables, fruits, a little meat and some seeds, but very little or no grain. Exposure to foods outside this range, including chemicals and additives, is purported to be a major cause of the prevalence of food allergies today. In addition, the work involved in providing sufficient food for survival legislated against overeating. The fact that food allergies are increasing nationwide, combined with the fact that the very foods that are to be avoided in this diet are among the most allergenic, lends weight to this theory. There is abundant anecdotal evidence that after only a few weeks on the Stone Age diet, allergy sufferers see a marked improvement in their symptoms, to the point that gradual reintroduction of some of the offending foods on a rotating basis is possible.

Nutritional deficiencies are a contributing cause to some of the suspected origins of allergies. For example, if you are unable to digest completely some of the foods you consume, you are at higher risk for leaky gut syndrome. If this is the case, correction of the underlying deficiencies is necessary before much improvement can be expected. Both for relief of symptoms and for correction of nutritional deficiencies, alternative practitioners suggest the following:

Vitamins and Minerals

- Vitamin A deficiency contributes to poor digestion. Because Vitamin A is fat-soluble and therefore can be stored in the body, supplement carefully to avoid overdose and toxicity.

- Pantothenic acid, a B vitamin, boosts adrenal function, which in turn strengthens the immune system.

- High doses of vitamin C can alleviate the inflammation associated with allergy symptoms, as well as strengthening the immune system in general. Side effects of excess vitamin C dosage, however, can occur when this water-soluble vitamin is excreted, leading to irritation of the urinary tract. Try to achieve a balanced dose.

- The mineral zinc is involved in the production of stomach acid, critical to proper digestion of your food and correction or avoidance of leaky gut syndrome.

Bioflavinoids

Bioflavinoids are a group of super-antioxidants found naturally in many of the same fruits and vegetables that contain vitamin C. Sometimes known as 'vitamin P', bioflavinoids are a relatively recent discovery in nutritional science, and have come to be recognized as some of the most powerful substances for nutritional health and anti-allergy found in nature. Of particular importance is quercetin. The best fruit sources of quercetin, as well as other flavinoids, are the deep, dark red and purple fruits. Red grapes, blueberries, red apples, red cherries and blackberries are all great sources. Even a glass of red wine will provide the body with a dose of protective antioxidants. Vegetable sources include broccoli, onion and green leafy vegetables all contain quercetin, as does red tea.

Bromelain, an enzyme found in pineapple, is both a synergistic booster for quercetin, helping with absorption, and on its own breaks up mucous and relieves inflammation.

Herbal Substances

Stinging nettle in capsule or tincture form is one of the most-recommended anti-allergy substances for its property of reducing allergic response. Other herbal remedies mentioned for various types of allergy are anticatarrhals like goldenseal, red sage, and goldenrod, which help eliminate mucus. In addition, astringents such as yarrow and myrrh (Commiphora myrrha) help contract inflamed tissues and reduce secretions and discharges. To strengthen immune response, Echinacea, astragalus root, goldenseal root, and Pfciffia paniculata (suma or Brazilian ginseng), a Brazilian herb that numerous studies have shown to be effective and safe for treating weakened immune systems. Use and dosage of these herbal substances as well as others too numerous to mention should be supervised by a naturopath or nutritionist well acquainted with their properties.

Other Treatments

Treatments not associated with medicines or vitamin or herbal therapy include alternative practices designed to increase or un-block energy flow, such as massage and acupuncture, and detoxification practices such as hydrotherapy and fasting, as well as some that are unproven at best. If you are suffering from allergies, have not been able to find relief with more conventional therapies and are considering some alternative method, be sure to research carefully to avoid practices that are ineffective and a waste of money at best and dangerous at worst.

Allergy Friendly Foods

With the exception, again, of foods that are cross-reactive with other allergens to which you have a known sensitivity, include the following foods in an allergy-friendly diet.

Bioflavinoid-rich Foods

- **Red Bell Peppers or Sweet Peppers** – According to some sources, red peppers contain three times more vitamin C than orange juice. Raw bell peppers are a safe and effective way to increase bioflavinoids in your diet.

- **Strawberries and other berries** are a great source of bioflavinoids. Claims of health benefits for berry-made wines and derivative foods are also prevalent. Just be sure that the derivative foods are not also highly processed or high in sugar.

- **Citrus Fruits** – Lemons, limes, peaches, nectarines and other fruits all contain vitamin C and bioflavonoid superoxidants, with oranges and grapefruit high on the list.

- **Broccoli** – A great source of vitamin C as well as some other essential vitamins, use it raw for best results.

- **Brussels sprouts** – Include these vegetables that are rich in antioxidants to get bioflavinoids and vitamins. If you have never enjoyed Brussels sprouts because you have always used the frozen variety, you are in for a treat if you will try fresh ones. Sweet, delicious and tender, they are great either steamed or seared in a skillet with caramelized onions. For the latter preparation, cut in half lengthwise and place facedown in the skillet in which you caramelized the onions, until lightly seared.

- **Tropical Fruits** – Exotic fruits, like mangoes and papayas, are becoming more accessible at supermarkets everywhere. Do not miss out on what they have to offer—a powerful punch of bioflavinoids.

- **Garlic** – We food culture have long been aware of garlic's anti-inflammatory properties, but now scientists are making this super food known as a natural food rich in bioflavinoids.

- **Spinach** – This green vegetable rich in antioxidants is a good all-purpose nutrient – try it in place of lettuce for a salad that is bursting with nutrition, or boost the nutrition of soups and stews with it.
- **Teas** – Green tea is known to have health benefits associated with bioflavinoids, and is generally caffeine-free. In addition, try red tea for quercetin, and even black tea has nutritional benefits.

In short, all the 'health' foods that pundits recommend are more often than not perfect for an anti-allergy diet.

Raw vs. Processed

As mentioned above in the Foods to Avoid section, highly processed foods have most of the beneficial nutrients removed in processing and are therefore nutritionally void if not frankly dangerous. Always bearing in mind that OAS would be an exception, your health, including allergy symptoms, will improve if you eat most fruits and vegetables raw rather than cooked. Always opt for the least processed of the choices you have in selecting a particular food, i.e. fresh rather than frozen, frozen over canned, whole-grain rather than refined.

Variety

Vary your food choices for better nutrition and avoidance of sensitization. Avoid eating any one food to the exclusion of all others or in excess (as in food addiction). Select foods according to the Stone Age diet; that is, the majority of your foods should be those prevalent among our Paleolithic ancestors. These included mostly fresh fruits and vegetables, fish and a little meat when it was available, along with some seeds. It definitely did NOT include processed grains or refined sugars.

This one practice alone will improve much more than your sensitivity to allergies; it will help regulate your blood sugar, reduce unhealthy stored fat, correct Candida yeast overgrowth, improve digestion to correct leaky gut syndrome and above all provide you with abundant energy.

More Books by John McArtur

You can visit John's author page at Amazon to see all his books.

http://www.amazon.com/John-McArthur/e/B001KMFW1O/

Hypothyroidism
Hypothyroidism: The Hypothyroidism Solution. Hypothyroidism Natural Treatment and Hypothyroidism Diet for Under Active Or Slow Thyroid, Causing Weight Loss Problems, Fatigue, Cardiovascular Disease. John McArthur (Author), Cheri Merz (Editor)

Fibromyalgia and Chronic Fatigue
Fibromyalgia And Chronic Fatigue: A Step-By-Step Guide For Fibromyalgia Treatment And Chronic Fatigue Syndrome Treatment. Includes Fibromyalgia Diet And Chronic Fatigue Diet And Lifestyle Guidelines. John McArthur (Author), Cheri Merz (Editor)

Yeast Infection
Candida Albicans: Yeast Infection Treatment. Treat Yeast Infections With This Home Remedy. The Yeast Infection Cure. John McArthur (Author)

Heart Disease
Hypertension - High Blood Pressure: How To Lower Blood Pressure Permanently In 8 Weeks Or Less, The Hypertension Treatment, Diet and Solution. John McArthur (Author)

Cholesterol Myth: Lower Cholesterol Won't Stop Heart Disease. Healthy Cholesterol Will. Cholesterol Recipe Book & Cholesterol

Diet. Lower Cholesterol Naturally Keep Cholesterol Healthy. John McArthur (Author), Cheri Merz (Editor)

Heart Disease Prevention and Reversal: How To Prevent, Cure and Reverse Heart Disease Naturally For A Healthy Heart . John McArthur (Author)

Diabetes
Diabetes Diet: Diabetes Management Options. Includes a Diabetes Diet Plan with Diabetic Meals and Natural Diabetes Food, Herbs and Supplements for Total Diabetes Control. Delicious Recipes. John McArthur (Author), Corinne Watson (Editor)

Diabetes Cooking: 93 Diabetes Recipes for Breakfast, Lunch, Dinner, Snacks and Smoothies. A Guide to Diabetes Foods to Help You Prepare Healthy Delicious ... Diabetic Meals and Natural Diabetes Food) John McArthur (Author), Corinne Watson (Editor)

Stress and Anxiety
From Stressful to Successful in 4 Easy Steps: Stress at Work? Stress in Relationship? Be Stress Free. End Stress and Anxiety. Excellent Stress Management, Stress Control and Stress Relief Techniques. John McArthur (Author)

Anxiety and Panic Attacks: Anxiety Management. Anxiety Relief. The Natural And Drug Free Relief For Anxiety Attacks, Panic Attacks And Panic Disorder. John McArthur (Author), Cheri Merz (Editor)

Back and Neck Pain
The 15 Minute Back Pain and Neck Pain Management Program: Back Pain and Neck Pain Treatment and Relief 15 Minutes a Day No Surgery No Drugs. Effective, Quick and Lasting Back and Neck Pain Relief. John McArthur (Author)

Arthritis

Arthritis: Arthritis Relief for Osteoarthritis, Rheumatoid Arthritis, Gout, Psoriatic Arthritis, and Juvenile Arthritis. Follow The Arthritis Diet, Cure and Treatment Free Yourself From The Pain. John McArthur (Author)

Depression

How to Break the Grip of Depression: Read How Robert Declared War On Depression ... And Beat It! John McArthur (Author)

Pregnancy

Pregnancy and Childbirth: Expecting a Baby. Pregnancy Guide. Pregnancy What to Expect. Pregnancy Health. Pregnancy Eating and Recipes. Cheri Merz (Author), John McArthur (Author)

Pregnancy Nutrition: Pregnancy Food. Pregnancy Recipes. Healthy Pregnancy Diet. Pregnancy Health. Pregnancy Eating and Recipes. Nutritional Tips and 63 Delicious Recipes for Moms-to-Be. Corinne Watson (Author), John McArthur (Author)

Allergies

Allergy Free: Fast Effective Drug-free Relief for Allergies. Allergy Diet. Allergy Treatments. Allergy Remedies. Natural Allergy Relief. John McArthur (Author), Cheri Merz (Editor)

Bibliography

1.   Encyclopedia of Natural Medicine Revised 2nd Edition: Michael Murray N.D. and Joseph Pizzorno N.D.

2.   Alternative Medicine: The Definitive Guide; Second Edition: Larry Trivieri, JR Editor, Introduced by Burton Goldberg.

3.   Alternative Cures: Bill Gottlieb

4.   How To Win The War Against Allergies: Wings of Success

5.   The Allergy Relief Sourcebook: AXXA Publishing

6.   Food Allergy - An Overview: National Institute of Allergy and Infectious Diseases: U.S. Department Of Health And Human Services